68

Tips

For Keeping Children Safe Inside & Outside the Home

FOR PARENTS, GRANDPARENTS,
BABY SITTERS,
TEACHERS, AND ANYONE
WHO OVERSEES CHILDREN

MURIEL ESSELL-CRENTSIL

About the Author

This book about injury prevention in children comes to you from the more than 20 years of expert experience of a former licensed family day care provider, registered nurse, health educator, and children's book author:
Muriel Essell-Crentsil, RN, BSN, BA

Prevention Saves Lives!

"Prevention must be our priority and our passion!"

Muriel Essell-Crentsil

General Safety Rules to Protect Your Children

- Call 911 or seek immediate medical attention, if a person is not breathing or has no pulse. Start cardiopulmonary resuscitation (CPR) if you are trained to do so. PREVENT DELAYS & SAVE LIVES.

- Buckle up children in an approved car seat; PREVENT INJURY OR DEATH IN CASE OF AN ACCIDENT.

- Always watch children in or near water; PREVENT DROWNING.

- Call the Poison Control Center if you think a child HAS BEEN POISONED

- HAVE AN EMERGENCY PLAN; make a list of emergency phone numbers, and post it in a visible location for all caregivers to see. *Example:* Post the list of emergency numbers on the refrigerator.

- Close and constant supervision of infants and children ARE THE BEST SAFETY BLANKETS.

Home Safety

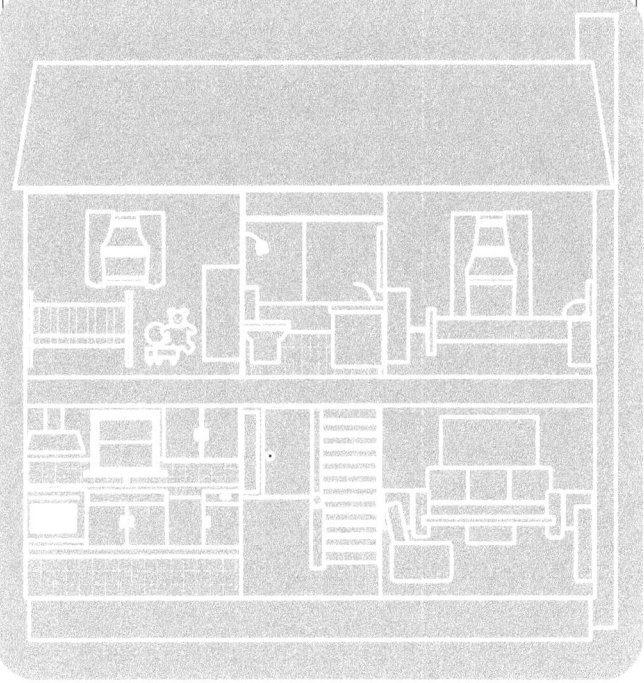

1.

Keep stairways clear and uncluttered.

PREVENT TRIPPING & FALLING

2.

Keep stairs and hallways well lit.

PREVENT FALLS

3.

Install safety gates at the top and bottom of stairs.

PREVENT FALLS

4.

Cover unused electric outlets with safety covers.

PREVENT ELECTROCUTION

5.

Install guards around fireplaces, radiators, wood burning stoves and hot pipes.

PREVENT BURNS

6.

Cushion the sharp edges of furniture with corner guards.

PREVENT INJURY

7.

Children have died when furniture tipped over on them. Secure furniture with anchors to the wall to prevent it from tipping over and falling.

PREVENT RISK OF INJURY AND DEATH

8.

Secure windows with
window locks.

PREVENT FALLS

9.

Keep plastic bags out of children's reach.

PREVENT CHOKING OR SUFFOCATION

10.

Install fire extinguishers
where they will be
most accessible.

TO PUT OUT FIRE IF NEEDED

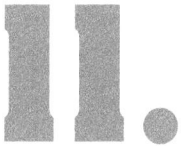

Install smoke detectors on each level of your home, outside sleeping areas and inside each bedroom and change the batteries at least twice a year.

GET ALERTS BEFORE A FIRE STARTS

12.

Install
carbon monoxide alarms
outside sleeping areas.

PREVENT CARBON
MONOXIDE POISONING

13.

Have an emergency escape plan to use in case of fire. (*Example:* Nearest exit door or window).

HAVE THE ENTIRE FAMILY PRACTICE THE PLAN OFTEN

14.

Set the hot water from the faucets at a safe temperature of 120° F.

PREVENT SCALDING

15.

Keep guns unloaded,
locked and
out of reach of children.

PREVENT DEATH OR SERIOUS INJURY

16.

Keep all purses, handbags and briefcases out of reach of children.

PREVENT KIDS FROM INGESTING OR SWALLOWING SMALL OBJECTS

17.

Keep all poisonous plants out of your child's reach.

PREVENT POISONING WHICH CAN BE FATAL

18.

For any family member or child with a health concern, post a list of instructions in a visible location for all caregivers to see.

KEEP MEDICATION LIST, ALLERGIES, & MEDICAL INSURANCE CARD NUMBER HANDY IN CASE OF AN EMERGENCY

19.

Keep a list of emergency phone numbers posted near a telephone or on a refrigerator.

**HAVE EASY ACCESS
IN AN EMERGENCY**

20.

Keep curtain cords
and shade pulls out of
a child's reach.

PREVENT STRANGULATION

Bathroom Safety

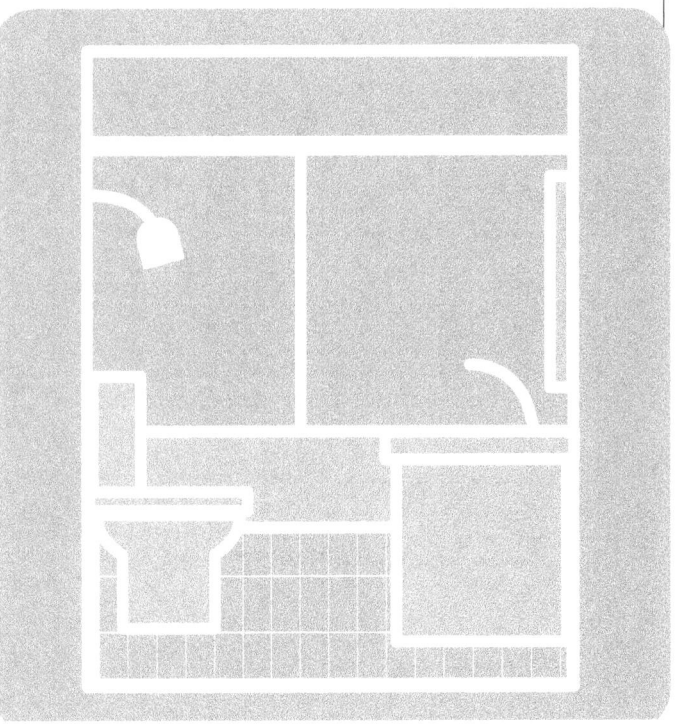

21.

Never leave a child
unattended
in the bathroom.
A child must always be
watched by an adult.

PREVENT DROWNING

22.

Secure cabinets with safety latches and keep them closed.

PREVENT CHILDREN FROM REACHING UNSAFE OBJECTS

23.

Keep all medicines
in child-resistant containers
and locked in a
medicine cabinet.

**PREVENT ACCIDENTAL
INGESTION OF MEDICINE
BY CHILDREN
WHICH COULD BE FATAL**

24.

Bottles of mouthwash, perfume, nail polish and nail polish remover must be stored out of reach of children.

THEY CAN BE FATAL IF SWALLOWED

25.

Keep razors and
other sharp objects out of
child's reach.

PREVENT INJURIES

26.

Store hair dryers, curling irons
and other electrical appliances
unplugged and away
from water
(sink, tub and toilet).

PREVENT BURNS OR
ELECTROCUTION

27.

Keep small objects out of
children's reach,
to prevent choking
if swallowed.
Keep button batteries
out of reach—they can be
poisonous.

PREVENT CHOKING
AND POISONING

28.

Use rubber stickers or a rubber mat on the floor of the tub or shower.

PREVENT SLIPS & FALLS

29.

Keep the toilet seat and lid down when the toilet is not in use.

PREVENT ACCIDENTAL DROWNING

Kitchen Safety

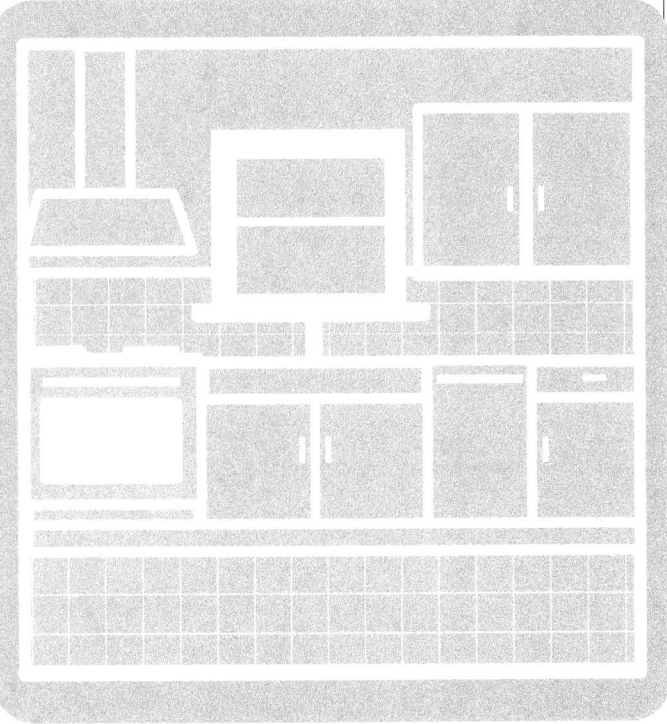

30.

Never leave baby alone in a
highchair and always
use all safety straps.

PREVENT INJURY

31.

Cook on the back burners
of the stove if children
are present.
Always turn pot handles
toward the back of the stove.

PREVENT BURNS

32.

Keep hot dishes away from
the edges of tables
and counter tops.

PREVENT BURNS

33.

Keep knives and other sharp objects out of the reach of children.

PREVENT CUTS & PUNCTURE WOUNDS

34.

Keep matches and lighters
out of the reach
of children.

PREVENTS BURNS
AND FIRES

35.

Place highchairs away
from a
stove and
other appliances.

PREVENT BURNS

36.

Keep all electrical appliances with cords (toasters, irons etc.) out of reach of children and unplugged to prevent burns, strangulation or electrocution.

AVOID BURNS & FALLING OBJECTS

37.

All cabinets must have
safety latches.

AVOID POISONING
BY CLEANING AGENTS

38.

Test the temperature of heated food before feeding a child.

PREVENT BURNS

39.

Keep all cabinet doors closed when not in use.

PREVENT EASY REACH OF INEDIBLES BY CHILDREN

40.

Keep cleaning products out of children's reach.

PREVENT ACCIDENTAL INGESTION

Child's Bedroom Safety

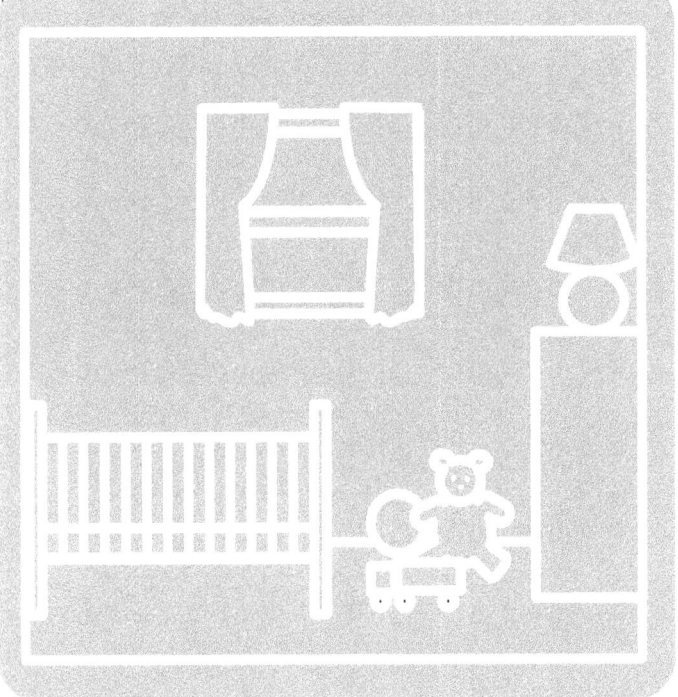

41.

Always lay babies
down to sleep on their back,
on a firm mattress,
and in a crib that meets
current safety standards.

PREVENT SUFFOCATION

42.

Avoid tummy sleeping.

PREVENT
SUDDEN INFANT DEATH
SYNDROME (SIDS)
AND SUFFOCATION

43.

If you use night-lights,
make sure they
are not touching
any fabric such as
bedspreads or curtains.

PREVENT FIRES

44.

Do not place babies to sleep on pillows or folded quilts.

PREVENT SUFFOCATION

45.

Do not use any crib with missing, broken, or loose parts. Make sure you tighten hardware from time to time to keep the crib sturdy.

PREVENT INJURY

46.

Place a child's bed or crib away from radiators and other hot surfaces.

PREVENT BURNS

47.

A crib mattress should
fit tightly.
(Gap around the mattress and
the side of the crib should be
less than two fingers).

PREVENT SUFFOCATION
& ENTRAPMENT

48.

Ensure that the paint and finish on baby furniture and toys are nontoxic.

PREVENT POISONING

49.

Keep electric cords out of child's reach and away from cribs.

PREVENT STRANGULATION OR ELECTROCUTION

50.

Child's clothing—especially sleepwear—must be flame resistant.

PREVENT BURNS

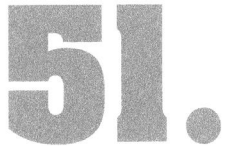

51.

A toy box must have a secure lid and safe closing hinges.

PREVENT EASY ACCESS TO TOYS THAT MAY CAUSE HARM

52.

Toys must be in good repair.

BROKEN TOYS MAY CAUSE INJURY TO A CHILD

53.

Toys must be appropriate
for a child's age.

TOYS WITH SMALL PARTS
MAY HARM A SMALL CHILD
IF SWALLOWED

54.

Remove all drawstrings from a child's clothing.

PREVENT STRANGULATION

55.

Keep toys with magnets away from young children. Two or more magnets, if swallowed, can attract through intestinal walls and cause holes, blockages and infection which can result in death.

PREVENT DEATH & INJURY

Parents' Bedroom Safety

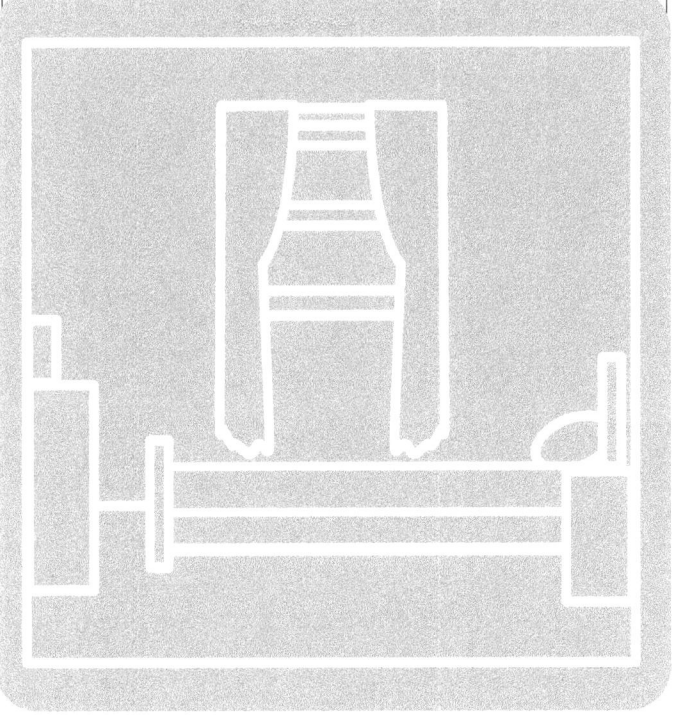

56.

Avoid using balloons around small children.

IF SWALLOWED, UNINFLATED BALLOONS AND BALLOON PIECES CAN CLING TO AIRWAYS AND LEAD TO DEATH

57.

Keep space heaters away from curtains and flammable materials.

PREVENT FIRES & BURN INJURIES

58.

Store cosmetics, perfumes
and breakable items
out of
children's reach.

PREVENT CHOKING,
POISONING AND INJURIES

59.

Keep small objects such as jewelry, buttons and safety pins out of children's reach.

PREVENT INJURY

MURIEL ESSELL-CRENTSIL

Outdoor & Playground Safety

60.

Keep trash in tightly covered containers.

PREVENT ACCIDENTAL INGESTION & UNWELCOME PESTS

61.

Keep walkways, stairs, and railings in good repair.

PREVENT FALLS AND INJURY

62.

Cover sandboxes and
wading pools
when not in use.

PREVENT ACCIDENTS
AND INJURY

63.

Make sure playground
equipment is safe
and assembled
according to the
manufacturer's instructions
and anchored
over soft surface such as
sand or wood chips.

PREVENT INJURY

64.

Wear a sun-protective hat
on sunny days.
Reduce ultraviolet radiation to
the face, head, and neck.

PREVENT SKIN CANCER

65.

Use insect repellants before going outdoors. Prevent bug bites and stings that could lead to severe and sometimes life threatening allergic reactions.

THE BITES OF MOSQUITOES, FLEAS, TICKS, BEES, HORNETS, YELLOW JACKETS, WASPS, FIRE ANTS AND SPIDERS CAN BE HARMFUL

66.

Standing water around your home, especially in a pool, pond, or sewage system, breeds bacteria and insects that can transmit potentially deadly diseases like malaria, encephalitis and parasites.

STAGNANT WATER ATTRACTS RATS, MICE, ROACHES & MOSQUITOES, VECTORS OF DISEASES AND INFECTION

67.

Get rid of old tires that can collect rain water and cans and bottles that can cause injury if rusted or broken.

PREVENT INJURIES AND INFECTIONS

68.

Cover pools when not in use and make sure there is a fence with a locked gate around your pool to prevent children from falling in.

PREVENT DROWNING

www.ingramcontent.com/pod-product-compliance
Lightning Source LLC
Chambersburg PA
CBHW071221280526
45787CB00002B/757